AWAKE
INTUBATION
(procedure in brief)

Dr. Pallab Kanti Nath

DEDICATION

To Department of Anesthesiology at Medical College, Kolkata, who taught me whatever I know of the subject today.

<u>AWAKE INTUBATION</u>

First intubation for providing anaesthesia was reported by *Dr. William Macewan* in 1878.

Preliminaries:

· Airway assessment

During the preoperative visit take a detailed history and physical examination to assess the difficulties that may come during the process and help in planning management.

· Psychological preparation

Starts from the preanaesthetic interview. Discuss in details the problems and the planned management strategy. Winning the patient's confidence and cooperation is particularly important during awake intubation.

Pharmacological preparation

Premedication:

To allay anxiety, provide a clear and dry airway, and prevent aspiration of gastric contents. Keep a running suction and difficult airway cart ready at hand along with resuscitation equipments and personals.

For anxiety: *Use of drugs is controversial because in most cases the procedure is done in patients with an anticipated difficult airway where conventional techniques at ventilation and/or intubation is already considered difficult and even a minor dose misappropriation of a respiratory depressant drug may lend up into an emergent situation, the way out from which may prove tricky and troublesome to the physician with an aggravated risk to the patient. A proper psychological counselling helps to reduce anxiety levels in most adults and ensure cooperation. However in spite of that some patients may still require some degree of pharmacological support to ensure smooth operation of the procedure. Here the basic principle is therefore to give small doses of drugs with short duration of action in titrated doses such that an unanticipated situation arising out of an overdose can be prevented and if such a situation still arises, can be managed easily and effectively. Some of the options are given below.*

· **Intravenous (IV) midazolam:** Give in slow increments of 20 to 40 µg/kg IV. (Maximum dose of 100 to 200 µg/kg). Dose can be repeated every 5 min till desired level of anxiolysis is obtained. Reversal agent Flumazenil should be available ready at hand for immediate administration in case of an inadvertent overt respiratory depression. Titration is done with a dose of 0.2mg IV every minute till desired effect is obtained.

· **Remifentanil** 0.05 to 0.5 µg/kg IV. (Reversal agent: naloxone 0.5-1mcg/kg every 3-5 mins till desired response.)

· **Dexmedetomidine:** alpha-2 adrenoceptor agonist—sedative, analgesic and anaesthetic-sparing effects. It produces sedation without affecting ventilation. Dexmedetomidine also has potent antisialogogue action. It is used in a loading dose of 1 µg/kg IV over 10 min, followed by a continuous infusion of 0.2–0.7 µg/kg/hour. (antagonist: Atipamezole)

Antisialogogue: *Glycopyrrolate (10 µg/kg IV)*

Ensures a relatively dry field that facilitates good visibility. A dry field also provides better quality of topical anaesthesia by allowing the local anaesthetic to act on the mucosal surfaces in appropriate concentration.

Vasoconstriction: For the highly vascular mucosa in the nose and nasopharynx when a nasal intubation is planned. *Phenylephrine nasal drops (0.25-0.5%)* along with lignocaine produces vasoconstriction as well as topical anaesthesia. Other vasoconstrictors include *0.025–0.05% oxymetazoline* nasal drops.

Combination of an H2-receptor blocker (eg. *Ranitidine*) with a prokinetic agent (*metoclopramide*): Helps in preventing aspiration of gastric contents. Addition of a non-particulate antacid (30 mL of 0.3 M sodium citrate solution) improves the degree of such protection.

Preparation of equipment and personnel

Difficult airway cart, running suction, resuscitation drugs, trained personals

· Monitoring

Should be individualised based on the patient and comorbidities.

Basic monitors: electrocardiograph, noninvasive blood pressure and pulse oximeter

Capnography: Patients with difficult airway should have a means of confirming proper location of the endotracheal tube.

Gold standard for confirming tracheal intubation is identification of the tracheal rings and carina beyond the tip of the endotracheal tube using flexible fibreoptic broncoscopy.

Clinical confirmation: seeing the endotracheal tube pass between the vocal cords/ misting and demisting of the endotracheal tube during expiration and inspiration/ five-point auscultation (both infraclavicular regions, both upper axillary regions and epigastrium) to confirm bilateral air entry over the chest and absence of gurgling sounds over the epigastrium.

PROCEDURE PROPER:

Which nerves to block?

- *Terminal branches of the ophthalmic and maxillary divisions of the trigeminal nerve supplying the nasal cavity and turbinates.*
- *The oropharynx and posterior one-third of the tongue supplied by the glossopharyngeal nerve.*
- *Branches of the vagus (Superior and recurrent laryngeal nerve) innervating the epiglottis and more distal airway structures.*

Nerve block options: Nebulisation/ infiltration/ topicalization

NEBULISATION:

Lidocaine 4% is added to a standard nebulizer with a face mask attached. The patient is asked to inhale the vapour deeply. Around 15-30 minutes are required to for achieving a reasonably good level of topical anaesthesia throughout the oropharynx and trachea.

Advantage: simple technique and more acceptable to the patient.

Disadvantage: Density of anaesthesia achieved is variable. Many patients will retain an intact cough reflex, which can make intubation technically challenging. Also, inhalation of local anaesthetic vapours can lead to central nervous system depression in patients whose mental status may already be depressed owing to other disease processes.

TOPICALIZATION:

For nasal intubation: The nasal mucosa is anaesthetised using two pledgets soaked in *4% topical lignocaine* introduced gently under vision as far as they will go. The first one is applied at a 45-degree angle to the hard palate to anaesthetise the sphenopalatine ganglion while the second is introduced parallel to the dorsal surface of the nose to block the anterior ethmoidal nerve.

Oral cavity: *2% lignocaine viscous* is swished around in the mouth for 5–10 min. *Lignocaine 10% spray* can be also used (Delivers 10 mg lignocaine per activation).

Spray as you go via flexible fibreoptic broncoscope: In this technique the operator can spray the local anaesthetic through the suction channel *(lidocaine 4%)*. A continuous flow of oxygen *(2–3 litres per min)* helps to maintain oxygenation while at the same time clears secretions away from the optical system of the fibrescope. When lignocaine is injected through the suction channel along with a flow of oxygen, the later creates a fine spray of local anaesthetic that gets deposited under vision over the structures distal to the fibrescope.

INFILTRATION:

Glossopharyngeal nerve block anaesthetises the posterior one-third of tongue and oropharynx and laryngopharynx up to the vallecula including the anterior surface of epiglottis. Advantage of the block is prevention of retching that often occurs when the posterior one-third of the tongue is lifted during laryngoscopy.

· **Intraoral approach:** mouth is opened and the tongue is anesthetized with topical anaesthetic (eg. *Lignocaine 10 spray*). Then a 3 and 1/3rd -in 22-gaugue needle is used to place 5 mL of 2% lignocaine submucosally at the at the base of the posterior tonsillar pillar (palatopharyngeal fold).

· **Peristyloid approach:** patient is placed supine and a line is drawn between the angle of the mandible and the mastoid process. Using deep pressure, styloid process is palpated just posterior to the angle of the jaw along this line, and the needle is seated against the styloid process. The needle is then withdrawn slightly and 5-7 mL of *2% lignocaine* is injected.

· *Both approaches involve deposition of local anaesthetic in close proximity to the carotid artery, and careful aspiration before injection is essential.*

Superior laryngeal nerve block: Branch of Vagus. Sensory supply—mucosa of larynx above the vocal cords. Motor supply—cricothyroid muscle.

Technique involves bilateral injections of local anaesthetic at the level of the greater cornu of the hyoid bone. The patient is placed supine with the head extended. After appropriate aseptic precautions the cornu of the hyoid bone is located below the angle of the mandible by palpating outward from the thyroid notch along the upper border of the thyroid cartilage until the greater cornu is encountered just superior to its posterolateral margin. The nondominant hand is used to displace the hyoid bone toward the side to be blocked. A 25-gauge needle is inserted until the lateral aspect of the greater cornu is contacted. The needle is slightly withdrawn and aspirated for air and blood and if negative, 2 mL of 2% lidocaine with or without epinephrine (1:200,000) is injected. Procedure is repeated on the other side as well.

Recurrent Laryngeal Nerve Block: Branch of vagus. *Sensory supply—larynx below the vocal cord.*

Sufficient blockade can be obtained using the inhalational technique.

Transtracheal block: The cricothyroid membrane is located in the midline of neck by palpating downwards from the thyroid prominence as a gap in the midline where the finger dips between the thyroid and the cricoids cartilage. After sterile skin preparation, the overlying skin is anesthetized by raising a small skin wheal of local anaesthetic. Then a 22- or 20-gauge needle mounted on a 10-mL syringe with 4mL of 4% lidocaine is inserted perpendicularly till air is aspirated indicating the needle's location in larynx. Local anaesthetic is injected rapidly and the needle is withdrawn.

Injection results in coughing and dispersal of the drug through the airways diffusely blocking the sensory nerve endings of the recurrent laryngeal nerve.

Prevention of drug toxicity

In any technique that employs a local anaesthetic solution, the anaesthesiologist should keep a close track of the total amount of local anaesthetic drug used to prevent inadvertent drug toxicity.

Dose calculation of LA: limit total dose within 3-5 mg/ kg (lignocaine)

ABOUT THE AUTHOR

Dr. Pallab Kanti Nath is an Anesthesiologist who currently practices in Kolkata, India.

For queries relating to the book, he can be contacted at
drpknath@gmail.com